前　言

请注意《国际中医临床实践指南青少年特发性脊柱侧凸症》（以下简称本指南）的某些内容可能涉及专利。本指南的发布机构不承担识别专利的责任。

本指南主要起草单位：北京以宗整脊医学研究院、广东省深圳市中医院、山东第一医科大学、广东省中山市中医院。

本指南参与起草单位：中国中医科学院望京医院、北京昌平区光明骨伤医院、北京昌平区中西医结合医院、广东省中医院、广东省佛山市中医院、广西国际壮医医院、广西梧州市第三人民医院、广西平南同安骨伤医院、北京电力医院、中日友好医院、河南省中医院、山东省立第三医院、甘肃省中医院、宁夏固原市中医院、北京中医药大学、山东中医药大学第二附属医院、山东省枣庄市新远大腰腿痛专科医院、上海中医药大学附属龙华医院、北京理工大学医院、天津中医药大学第一附属医院、上海交通大学、浙江中医药大学、浙江省台州市路桥医院、广西中医药大学、贵州中医药大学附属医院、辽宁中医药大学附属第二医院、暨南大学附属第一医院、香港大学专业进修学院、美国纽约健康学院、德国艾森大学 AMC 医院、新西兰李氏中医研究院、俄罗斯伊尔库茨克中医院、马来西亚柔佛州针灸骨伤学会、澳大利亚中国中医针灸医疗研究院、加拿大中医学院、韩国推拿医学会、中国台湾台中市中医医院。

本指南主要起草人：韦以宗、林远方、师彬、陈世忠、王秀光、韦春德、郑晓斌、孙国栋。

本指南参与起草审阅人（按姓氏笔画排序）

中国：王松、王世轩、王慧敏、韦东德、邓强、石玉生、田新宇、冯华山、吕立江、闫固林、江智宏（台湾）、祁俊丽、孙胜林、李建军、李俊杰、李雄文、吴宁、应有荣、沈骏、张国仪（香港）、张盛强、陈栋、陈文治、陈连勇、陈德军、周霞、周红海、单衍丽、赵帅、赵勇、赵道洲、高腾、黄俊卿、梁树勇、梁倩倩、谭明生、潘东华、薛卫国。

美国：Josrph Sing Cheung、宋阿丽。

新西兰：李蔷薇。

韩国：申秉澈。

马来西亚：陈联国、苏圣仁。

加拿大：汤耿民。

德国：Jurgen Bachmann。

俄罗斯：李庆和。

澳大利亚：黄焕松。

本指南的起草，遵守了世界中医药学会联合会发布的《世界中医药学会联合会国际组织标准管理办法》和 SCM 0001－2009《标准制定和发布工作规范》。

本指南由世界中医药学会联合会发布，版权归世界中医药学会联合会所有。

引　言

为适应中医药国际化的发展趋势和要求，促进中医医师管理的规范化建设，提高国际中医师队伍的学术地位和整体素质，保障其合法权益，提高社会认可度，保证中医医疗质量和医疗安全，特制定本指南。

本指南的制定，既重视与世界各国医师管理法律法规相协调，又充分反映中医专业技术人员诊疗规律；既考虑世界各国中医药专业技术人员的现实情况，又有利于未来国际中医医师队伍的健康发展；既注重与国际中医医疗市场需求相适应，又有利于中医药学术发展和事业发展。

本指南在分析各国医师使用医学专业技术诊疗成功经验的基础上，从前瞻性地引领和规范国际中医医师诊疗的视角，科学、合理地确定了疾病规律和相关指标体系。

本指南的制定和实施，旨在为各国中医诊疗本病提供参考，不断提高中医师的服务能力和诊疗水平，保证中医医疗服务的安全性和质量，更好地为世界各国人民的健康服务。

本指南的制定和实施的根据是中医整脊学研究发现青少年特发性脊柱侧凸症源自腰大肌一侧不作为（萎缩性脂肪样变）及临床经验。

请注意，本指南的发布机构声明符合本指南时，可能涉及"整脊调曲牵引床"相关专利的使用。本指南的发布机构对于该专利的真实性、有效性和范围无任何立场。

该专利持有人已向本指南发布机构保证，愿意同任何申请人在合理且无歧视的条款和条件下，就专利授权许可进行谈判。该专利持有人的声明已在本指南的发布机构备案。

相关信息可以通过以下联系方式获得：

专利持有人姓名：韦以宗。

地址：北京市昌平区水库路朝凤山庄 8501 宅。

国际中医临床实践指南青少年特发性脊柱侧凸症

1 范围

本指南规定了青少年特发性脊柱侧凸症的术语与定义、诊断、辨证、治疗等内容。

本指南适用于 Cobb 角 40°以内、年龄 18 岁以下青少年特发性脊柱侧凸症的诊断和治疗。

2 规范性引用文件

本指南无规范性引用文件。

3 术语和定义

下列术语和定义适用于本指南。

青少年特发性脊柱侧凸症

年龄在 7 岁以上，出现脊柱的一个或数个节段在冠状面上向一侧隆凸和椎体旋转，并随年龄增长弯曲增大至发育成熟，而无任何先天性脊柱骨结构异常的疾病。

注 1：亦称"青少年特发性脊柱侧弯症"，属中医"小儿龟背"范畴。

注 2：该病多发于女性，男女比例为 1∶4 左右，常见于 7 至 14 岁青少年。

4 诊断

4.1 临床表现

4.1.1 症状

轻度的脊柱侧凸患者可以毫无症状，特别好发于青春期女性，随着月经来潮，侧凸逐年加大，至 18 岁发育成熟时停止。胸部及腰背部较少裸露，轻度畸形不易发现。多数是体检或沐浴更衣时被发现，多伴有肩胛高低不对称、腰部侧凸，可见凹陷侧肌肉瘦小、凸起侧丰隆、左右不对称。重度脊柱侧凸患者多伴有腰背疼痛、易疲劳、运动后气短、胸闷、心悸、下肢麻木等症状。

4.1.2 体征

患者脊柱呈侧凸畸形（棘突连线偏离中轴线）；脊柱两侧肌肉不对称；凹侧皮温可异常；两肩、两肩胛、两侧髂嵴不等高，严重者可出现驼背畸形、骨盆不对称、下肢不等长、步态倾斜。Adam 前屈试验阳性。

4.1.3 影像学和辅助检查及诊断分型

青少年特发性脊柱侧凸症的影像学和辅助检查及诊断分型参见附录 A。

4.2 鉴别诊断

4.2.1 继发性脊柱侧凸症

本症为因骨盆倾斜或椎间盘突出、椎间盘炎、骨肿瘤、骨结核、癔症、代谢性骨病、感染性骨病、外伤等其他疾病刺激引起的脊柱继发性侧凸。这种脊柱侧凸均能找到原发疾病，按原发疾病治疗，侧凸可改善或消失。

4.2.2 先天性脊柱侧凸症

本症为因先天性脊椎骨畸形导致的脊柱侧凸。此类侧凸自出生开始就出现。

5 辨证

5.1 肾阳亏虚证

脊柱呈侧凸畸形，多伴有坐久后腰部隐隐作痛，酸软无力，肢冷，喜暖，舌质淡，脉沉无力。

5.2 脾肾阳虚证

脊柱呈侧凸畸形，多伴有坐久后腰部隐隐作痛，酸软无力，肢冷，喜暖，纳差，倦怠懒言，气短乏力，大便稀溏，舌质淡红，舌苔滑腻，脉沉无力，或沉迟。

5.3 肾虚血瘀证

脊柱侧凸畸形日久，肌肤甲错，易劳累，舌质紫红，苔薄白，脉细涩。

6 治疗

6.1 治疗原则

以理筋、调曲、练功为主。

6.2 治疗方法

6.2.1 理筋疗法

6.2.1.1 药熨或熏蒸法

应用疏风散寒、通络药物,水煎后熨烫萎缩侧肌肉,或用药物蒸汽熏蒸萎缩侧肌肉,以促进萎缩肌肉恢复,每次30分钟。

6.2.1.2 针刺法

取脊柱凹侧华佗夹脊穴为主,以改善肌肉功能,每次30分钟。可加电针。

6.2.1.3 推拿、捏脊法

沿脊柱凹侧自腰骶开始捏拿皮肤和肌肉,捏脊松筋,以强健脾胃,配合肌肉萎缩侧擦、拿、揉、拍打等推拿、按摩手法,以恢复竖脊肌、腰方肌、髂腰肌肌力平衡。

6.2.2 正骨调曲疗法

6.2.2.1 正脊骨法

坐位行胸腰旋转法、腰椎旋转法及过伸提胸法,纠正椎体旋转,进而改善侧凸(正脊骨法具体操作方法及适应证、禁忌证、注意事项参见附录B)。

6.2.2.2 牵引调曲法

根据患者侧凸类型,应用整脊调曲牵引床,辨证行四维调曲法治疗,以调椎体旋转、侧凸,恢复脊柱生理曲度(牵引调曲法操作方法及适应证、禁忌证、注意事项参见附录B)。

上述理筋、调曲疗法每日1次,10次为1个疗程,休息1日,再行第2个疗程,一般治疗4~6个疗程。

6.2.3 药物疗法

6.2.3.1 分证论治

6.2.3.1.1 肾阳亏虚证

治法:补肾壮阳。

主方:右归丸(《景岳全书》)加减。

6.2.3.1.2 脾肾阳虚证

治法:温补脾肾。

主方:肾气丸(《伤寒论》)合附子理中丸(《伤寒论》)加减。

6.2.3.1.3 肾虚血瘀证

治法:补肾,活血化瘀。

主方:膈下逐瘀汤(《医林改错》)加减。

6.2.3.2 外用药

选用中医传统膏药,敷贴胸、腰凹侧,以利于活血化瘀,改善循环,恢复肌力。可用"千山活血膏"(国药准字 Z20025596)局部外贴。具体使用见该膏药说明。

6.2.3.3 其他药物疗法

可配合改善骨代谢及内分泌药物。

6.2.4 练功疗法

选用"健脊强身十八式"中的第六式、第十三式、第十四式及第十五式进行功能锻炼,加强腰背肌及腰大肌功能,以增强其活力和韧性,维护脊柱内外平衡(图1)。

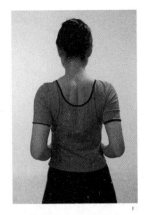

第六式：双胛合拢式：
扩胸，纠正胸椎侧凸

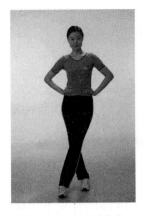

第十三式：剪步转盆式：
凸侧下肢在前，纠正骨盆旋转

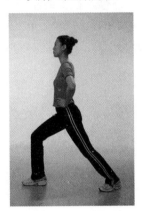

第十四式：前弓后箭式：
凸侧下肢在前，纠正腰椎旋转

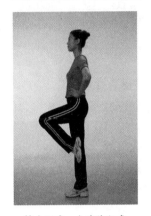

第十五式：金鸡独立式：
凸侧下肢屈曲，激活腰大肌

图 1   "健脊强身十八式"中的第六式、第十三式、第十四式及第十五式

6.3   疗效评估

疗效评估可分为如下四个等级：

——优：侧凸改善超过 30% 者。

——良：侧凸改善在 10% ~29% 者。

——差：侧凸改善不足 10% 者。

——无效：侧凸无改善者。

6.4   注意事项

6.4.1   前弓后箭式，注意凸侧下肢在前、凹侧下肢在后。

6.4.2   药熨、针灸、推拿均以肌肉萎缩侧为主进行治疗。

6.4.3   药熨时温度以患者适应为宜，不能过烫，避免烫伤；所用药物尽量选择对皮肤刺激小的，熨后如局部皮肤有红点、出现过敏反应者，需停用本法。

6.5   禁忌证

正脊骨法以旋转法为主，切忌暴力。

附　录　A

（资料性附录）

青少年特发性脊柱侧凸症检查及诊断分型

A.1　青少年特发性脊柱侧凸症检查

A.1.1　X线检查

脊柱正立位可见部分棘突偏离正中线，脊柱向一侧或两侧凸，部分椎间隙左右不等，椎体倾斜，椎体两侧不等高，可用Cobb法测量其具体侧凸角度。侧位可见颈、胸、腰生理曲度异常。

Cobb法：在正位X线摄片上，先确定侧凸的上终椎及下终椎，在主弯上、下两端其上、下终板线向凹侧倾斜度最大者，主弯上端者为上终椎，主弯下端者为下终椎。在上终椎椎体上缘及下终椎椎体下缘各画一平线，对此两横线各做一条垂直线，两条垂线的交角即为Cobb角，用量角器可测出具体度数。如果终椎上、下缘不清者，可取其椎弓根上下缘的连线，然后取其垂线的交角即为Cobb角。

A.1.2　脊柱CT三维立体重建

可清楚发现骨发育异常。

A.1.2　辅助检查

辅助检查包括测身高、体重、双臂外展位双中指尖间距等有关项目。被检查者裸露整个腰背部，自然站立，双足与双肩等宽，双目平视，手臂自然下垂，掌心向内。检查者站在其正后方，观察被检查者双肩是否对称，两侧髂嵴是否等高，棘突连线是否偏离中轴。五项中如有一项不正常便可诊为躯干不对称。

A.2　诊断分型

根据侧凸主曲线顶点的解剖位置，结合临床，将青少年特发性脊柱侧凸症分为以下三种类型。

A.2.1　I型

胸椎单弧型：主弧由胸椎组成，腰椎侧凸不明显。侧凸程度及预后有很大不同，弧度可发展到很严重，由于椎体旋转使胸椎后凸变平，肋骨后隆，而使肺功能下降，出现胸闷、气短等相应症状。肋骨后隆起的程度不一定与侧凸角度相称（图A.1）。

腰椎单弧型：主弧由腰椎组成，胸椎侧凸不明显，但会引起上半身向侧方倾斜（图A.2）。

A.2.2　II型

胸腰椎双弧型：胸椎弧顶点在胸7节段，并突向右侧，腰椎弧顶点在腰1～2节段，胸椎、腰椎侧凸同时发生，弯度也大体相同，凸侧肩胛肋骨隆起，椎体向凸侧的对侧旋转。胸腰椎弧度交界处的移行椎体无旋转畸形。在青少年时期侧凸有发展趋势（图A.3）。

A.2.3　III型

颈胸腰三弧型：颈胸段、胸段和腰段均出现侧凸（图A.4）。

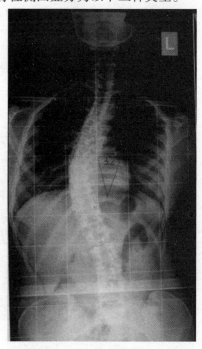

图A.1　侧凸胸椎单弧型

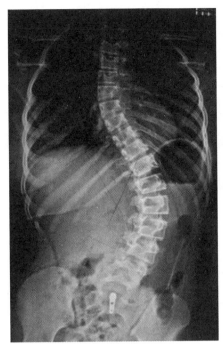

图 A.2 侧凸腰椎单弧型

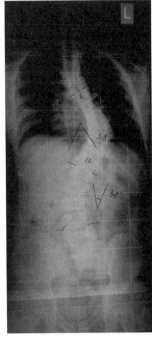

图 A.3 侧凸双弧型

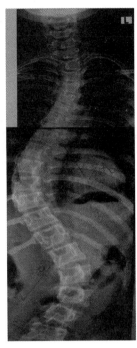

图 A.4 侧凸三弧型

附　录　B

（资料性附录）

常用正脊手法和牵引调曲法

B.1　提胸过伸法

B.1.1　适应证

提胸过伸法的适应证包括合并胸椎侧凸的各类颈椎病、脊柱侧凸症、脊椎骨骺软骨病、脊源性心律紊乱症、脊源性胃肠功能紊乱症。

B.1.2　禁忌证

严重骨质疏松患者禁用。

B.1.3　注意事项

膝顶法向前顶力不能过大。

B.1.4　操作方法

［术式一］患者骑坐在整脊椅上，面向前，双手十指交叉抱项部。医者站在患者后方，用一膝顶上段胸椎，双手自患者肩上伸向两侧胁部，然后双手抱两胁将患者向后上方提拉。

［术式二］患者骑坐在整脊椅上，面向前，双手十指交叉抱项部。医者站在患者背后，双手自患者腋下穿过，向上反握其双前臂，用前胸顶患者背部，然后双手用力，将患者向后上方提拉。

［术式三］患者骑坐在整脊椅上，面向前，双臂于前胸交叉，双手抱肩。医者坐在患者背后，从腋下双手拉患者对侧肘关节，使肩胛拉开，然后将患者向后上方提拉。

B.2　胸腰旋转法

B.2.1　适应证

胸腰旋转法的适应证包括胸腰椎小关节紊乱、腰椎滑脱症、腰椎间盘突出症、腰椎管狭窄症、脊柱侧凸症、脊源性月经紊乱症、脊源性下肢骨性关节炎、脊源性胃肠功能紊乱症、强直性脊柱炎脊柱畸形症。

B.2.2　禁忌证

胸腰旋转法的禁忌证包括胸腰椎手术后、腰椎严重骨质疏松、胸腰椎骨肿瘤、胸腰椎骨结核、胸腰椎骨髓炎。腰椎间盘突出症急性期及腰僵未缓解者慎用。

B.2.3　注意事项

施法时需有助手固定髋部。忌为强求响声，反复旋转。

B.2.4　操作方法

患者骑坐在整脊椅上，面向前，双手交叉抱后枕部，略向前屈至以胸12或腰1为顶点。以棘突左偏为例，助手固定患者右髋，医者立于患者左侧后方，左手经过患者左臂前，至颈胸背部（大椎以下），右手固定于胸腰枢纽关节左侧，左手旋转患者胸腰部，待患者放松后，双手相对同时用力，即左手向左旋转的同时右手向右推，可听到局部"咯嗒"声。右侧操作与左侧相反。

B.3　腰椎旋转法

B.3.1　适应证

腰椎旋转法的适应证包括腰椎后关节错缝症、腰骶后关节病、腰椎间盘突出症、腰椎管狭窄症、腰椎侧凸症。

B.3.2　禁忌证

B.3.2.1　同胸腰枢纽旋转法禁忌证。

B.3.2.2 椎间盘突出压迫硬脊膜囊大于1/2者禁用。

B.3.2.3 椎弓崩解、脊柱滑脱者慎用。

B.3.3 注意事项

同胸腰旋转法。

B.3.4 操作方法

患者骑坐在整脊椅上，面向前，双手交叉抱后枕部，向前屈至棘突偏歪处为顶点。以棘突左偏为例，助手固定右髋，医者立于患者左侧后方，左手穿过患者左腋下至对侧肩部，右手掌固定于偏歪棘突左侧，左手摇动患者腰部，待患者放松后，双手相对同时瞬间用力，即左手向左旋转的同时右手向右推，可听到局部"咯嗒"声。右侧操作与左侧相反。

B.4 四维调曲法

B.4.1 适应证

B.4.1.1 屈曲型胸腰椎骨折脱位。

B.4.1.2 腰椎曲度变直、反弓的腰椎间盘突出症。

B.4.1.3 腰椎曲度变直、反弓的腰椎管狭窄症。

B.4.1.4 腰椎曲度变直、反弓的腰椎后关节错缝症。

B.4.1.5 脊柱侧凸症。

B.4.1.6 腰椎曲度变直、反弓或上弓下曲的腰椎滑脱症。

B.4.2 禁忌证

B.4.2.1 诊断不明确，未具备X线摄片诊断骨关节力学改变者。

B.4.2.2 腰椎间盘突出症急性期牵引后疼痛加重者。

B.4.2.3 合并严重高血压、心脏病、哮喘及甲亢者。

B.4.2.4 孕妇及严重骨质疏松患者。

B.4.2.5 腰椎手术后患者。

B.4.2.6 脊柱骨结核、脊柱骨髓炎、脊柱骨肿瘤、严重下肢骨性关节病、严重静脉曲张患者。

B.4.3 操作方法

患者卧于整脊调曲牵引床上，将上半身用环套过腋下，双下肢牵引带束于膝关节上、下端。用

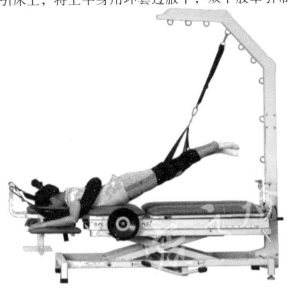

图 B.1 四维牵引（俯卧过伸悬吊牵引）拉伸腰大肌等长收缩

升降板将下半身托起，升降板的胸腰段与上半身呈 25°～45°角（图 B.1），调整牵引仪，使双下肢缓慢升起，下半身呈悬吊状，后将托板放至离下肢约 30cm 处，以下腹部离开托板为宜。下肢与牵引床的角度根据患者腰椎曲度进行调整，一般情况下力的支点作用在胸腰枢纽关节处。牵引时间为 20～30 分钟，以患者耐受为度。牵引解除后，卧床休息 10～20 分钟方可下地。

B.4.4 注意事项

B.4.4.1 束于下肢的带子不能固定在髌骨上，而且要松紧适度，不能太紧，以免影响血液循环。

B.4.4.2 双下肢悬吊需逐步升高，并随时观察患者病情变化。

B.4.4.3 牵引时间以患者耐受为度，逐渐增加牵引时间。

B.4.4.4 牵引时密切观察患者足背动脉搏动情况。

B.4.4.5 撤除牵引时要匀速、缓慢，解开下肢牵引带后缓慢将托板放下。

Foreword

It is noted that there may be some issues associated with patent. The agency publishing *International Guidelines for Clinical Practice of Traditional Chinese Medicine Adolescent Idiopathic Scoliosis* (hereinafter referred to as guideline) declares that no responsibility is taken for recognizing these patents.

The main drafting institutes of this "guideline": Beijing Yizong Institute of Spinal Orthopedics in Chinese Medicine, Guangdong Shenzhen Hospital of Traditional Chinese Medicine, Shandong First Medical University (Shandong Academy of Medical Sciences), Guangdong Zhongshan Hospital of Traditional Chinese Medicine.

The following institutes have completed the drafting of this guideline: Wangjing Hospital of Chinese Academy of Traditional Chinese Medicine. Beijing Changping District Bright Bone Injury Hospital. Beijing Changping District Hospital of Integrated Traditional Chinese and Western Medicine. Guangdong Hospital of Traditional Chinese Medicine. Foshan Hospital of Traditional Chinese Medicine, Guangdong Province. Guangxi International Zhuang Medical Hospital. Guangxi Wuzhou the Third People's Hospital. Guangxi Pingnan Tongan Bone Injury Hospital. Beijing Electric Power Hospital. China – Japan Friendship Hospital. Henan Hospital of Traditional Chinese Medicine. Shandong Provincial Third Hospital. Gansu Provincial Hospital of Traditional Chinese Medicine. Ningxia Guyuan Hospital of Traditional Chinese Medicine. Beijing University of Traditional Chinese Medicine. The Second Affiliated Hospital of Shandong University of Traditional Chinese Medicine. Shandong Province Zaozhuang Xinyuanda Lumbago Specialist Hospital. Longhua Hospital Affiliated to Shanghai University of Traditional Chinese Medicine. Beijing Institute of Technology Affiliated Hospital. The First Affiliated Hospital of Tianjin University of Traditional Chinese Medicine. Shanghai Jiao Tong University. Zhejiang University of Chinese Medicine. Luqiao Hospital, Taizhou City, Zhejiang Province. Guangxi University of Traditional Chinese Medicine. Affiliated Hospital of Guizhou University of Traditional Chinese Medicine. The Second Affiliated Hospital of Liaoning University of Traditional Chinese Medicine. The First Affiliated Hospital of Jinan University. Faculty of Continuing and Professional Studies, University of Hong Kong. New York Medical College. AMC Hospital, Eisen University, Germany. Lee's Institute of Traditional Chinese Medicine, New Zealand. Irkutsk Hospital of Traditional Chinese Medicine, Russia. Malaysia Johor Institute of Bone Injury and Acupuncture. Australian Chinese Medicine Acupuncture Medical Research Canadian College of Traditional Chinese Medicine. Korean Massage Medical Association. Taichung Hospital of Traditional Chinese Medicine, Taiwan, China.

The main drafters of this guideline: Wei Yizong. Lin Yuanfang. Shi Bin. Chen Shizhong. Wang Xiuguang. Wei Chunde. Zheng Xiaobin. Sun Guodong.

The participating drafters of this guideline: (sorted by stroke of surname): China: Wang Song. Wang Shixuan. Wang Huimin. Wei Dongde. Deng Qiang. Shi Yusheng. Tian Xinyu. Feng Huashan. Lv Lijiang. Yan Gulin. Jiang Zhihong (Taiwan). Qi JunLi. Sun Shenglin. Li Jianjun. Li Junjie. Li Xiongwen. Wu Ning. Ying Yourong. Shen Jun. Zhang Guoyi (Hong Kong). Zhang Shengqiang. Chen Dong. Chen Wenzhi. Chen Lianyong. Chen Dejun. Zhou Xia. Zhou Honghai. Chan YanLi. Zhao Shuai. Zhao Yong. Zhao Daozhou. Gao Teng. Huang Junqing. Liang Shuyong. Liang Qianqian. Tan Mingsheng. Pan Donghua. Xue

Weiguo.

America: Josrph Sing Cheung. Song Ali.

New Zealand: Li Qiangwei.

South Korea: Shen Bingche.

Malaysia: Chen Lianguo. Su Shengren.

Canada: Tang Gengmin.

Germany: Jurgen Bachmann.

Russia: Li Qinghe.

Australia: Huang Huansong.

The drafting of this guideline complies with *International Organization Standard Management method of World Federation of Chinese Medicine Societies* and SCM 0001 – 2009 *Standard Formulation and Issuance Work Specification* issued by World Federation of Chinese Medicine Societies.

This guideline is issued and copyrighted by the World Federation of Chinese Medicine Societies.

Introduction

In order to adapt to the development trend of internationalization of traditional Chinese medicine and requirements, promote the construction of TCM physicians and the standardization of the management, improve the academic status and the overall quality of the contingent of international TCM physicians, protect their legitimate rights and interests, increase social recognition, guarantee medical quality and medical safety of traditional Chinese medicine, this guideline is established.

The formulation of this guideline should not only pay attention to the coordination with the laws and regulations on the management of doctors in various countries, but also fully reflect the rules of diagnosis and treatment for TCM professionals. The guideline should not only take into account the actual situation of TCM professionals in various countries, but also be conducive to the healthy development of the international team of TCM doctors in the future. It should not only meet the needs of the international TCM medical market, but also be conducive to the academic and career development of TCM.

Based on the analysis of the successful experience in the diagnosis and treatment of doctors in various countries, this guideline leads and standardizes the diagnosis and treatment of international TCM doctors from a prospective perspective, which is scientific. The rule of disease and relative index system were determined reasonably.

The formulation and implementation of this guideline can provide reference for the TCM diagnosis and treatment of diseases in various countries. It will continue to improve the service capabilities and diagnosis and treatment of TCM physicians, ensure the safety and quality of TCM medical service, and serve the health of people better around the world.

The formulation and implementation of this guideline is based on the research of literature referring to Chinese chiropractic, which found that adolescent specific scoliosis originated from the inaction of one side of psoas major muscle (atrophic lipomatosis), and was formulated according to clinical experience.

The patent holder has assured with the agency publishing this document that, under reasonable and non – discriminatory principles, he is willing to negotiate the issue about patent and license with any applicant. The statement of the patent holder has been registered in the agency publishing this guideline.

This guideline relates to the patent number ZL03261021. 1 of "Chiropractic tune traction bed" Chinese utility model, the patent holder is Wei Yizong, and the address is 8501 House, Chaofeng Mountain Villa, Shuiku Road, Changping District, Beijing.

International Guidelines for Clinical Practice of Traditional Chinese Medicine Adolescent Idiopathic Scoliosis

1 Scope

This guideline provides the term and definition, diagnosis, syndrome differentiation and treatment of adolescent idiopathic scoliosis.

This guideline is applicable to the diagnosis and treatment of adolescent idiopathic scoliosis that the patient is younger than 18 years old with cobb angle being within 40 degrees.

2 Normative citation documents

There is no normative citation documents in this guideline.

3 Terms and definitions

The following terms and definitions are applied to this guideline.

Adolescent idiopathic scoliosis

Idiopathic scoliosis in adolescents means that after the age of 7 years, one or more segments of the spine appear to rotate sideways in the coronal plane(one side bulges and the vertebral body rotates), and the curvature increases with increasing age, without any congenital spine and bone structure abnormal.

Note 1: Adolescent idiopathic scoliosis belongs to the category of "pediatric turtle back" in Chinese medicine.

Note 2: This disease is often occurred in female. The proportion of male to female is 1 : 4, it is often seen in the adolescent aged 7 to 14.

4 Diagnosis

4.1 Diagnosis points

4.1.1 Symptoms

Patients with mild scoliosis sometimes have no symptoms. It especially prone to appear in adolescent women with menstrual tide, increased scoliosis year by year, until to the age of 18 years old that the mature development stops. The abnormal is hard to be found since the chest and lumbar part is rarely to be seen. Most physical conditions are discovered during a physical examination or during a shower or dressing. More with the height of the scapular asymmetry, lumbar scoliosis, visible thin sunken side muscles, convex side plump, left and right asymmetry. Patients with severe scoliosis have back pain, fatigue, shortness of breath after exercise, chest tightness, palpitations, numbness of the lower limbs and other symptoms.

4.1.2 Signs

The patient's spine is deformed (the spinous process line deviates from the central axis); the muscles on the two sides of the spine are asymmetric; the concave skin temperature is abnormal; The scapulae and iliac crest are asymmetrical. The sever patients appear humpback deformity, pelvis asymmetrical, the lower limbs with different length, and inclined walking posture . Adam forward bend test is positive.

4.1.3 Imaging and accessory inspection and diagnostic typing

They are the same as the appendix A.

4.2 Differential diagnosis

4.2.1 Secondary scoliosis

Secondary scoliosis caused by pelvic tilt or disc herniation, disc herniation, bone tumors, bone tuberculosis, hysteria, metabolic bone disease, infectious bone disease, trauma and other diseases stimulated. This scoliosis can always find the primary disease. Symptoms can be improved or disappeared according to the treatment of the primary disease.

4.2.2 Congenital scoliosis

Congenital scoliosis is due to congenital bone or spinal deformity, which occurs from birth, and there is no effective treatment.

5 Syndrome differentiation

5.1 Kidney yang deficiency syndrome

There is scoliosis malformation. Most of the patients have back lumber part pain after sitting for a long time, weakness, cold limbs and prefer warmth. The tongue is red, the fur is thin and white, the pulse is weak.

5.2 Spleen – kidney yang deficiency syndrome

There is scoliosis malformation. Most of the patients have back lumber part pain after sitting for a long time, weakness, cold limbs, poor appetite, fatigue, tiredness, lethargy, shortness of breath, loose stools, and prefer warmth. The tongue is slippery, the pulse is heavy and weak or slow and sunken.

5.3 Kidney deficiency and blood stasis syndrome

When suffering from scoliosis deformity for a long time, the patient's skin will be strained, and the patient is easily tired. The tongue is purplish red with thin white coating. The pulse is fine and astringent.

6 Treatment

6.1 Principles of treatment

Focusing on therapeutic manipulation for tendons, curvature adjustment and doing exercises.

6.2 Treatment methods

6.2.1 Tendon therapy

6.2.1.1 Medicinal ironing or fumigation

Decocting the relieving wind – cold syndrome andremoving obstruction in collaterals drugs oiron the atrophic side muscles with the drug or use the drug vapor to fumigate the atrophic side muscles to promote the recovery of atrophic muscles, 30 minutes each time.

6.2.1.2 Acupuncture

Take the Huatuo Jiaji points on the concave side of the spine as the treatment points to improve the muscle function, 30 minutes each time. An electric needle treatment can be used as an extra.

6.2.1.3 Massage and Chiropractic

Pinch and grasp the skin and muscles of the concave side of the spine from the lumbosacral region, for strengthening the spleen and stomach. and cooperate with massage techniques such as rolling, holding, kneading, and Quadratus erectus, quadratus psoas, iliopsoas tapping the muscle atrophy to restore muscle balance of erector spinae, quadratus lumborum, iliopsoas.

6.2.2 Orthopedic curvature adjusting therapy

6.2.2.1 Orthopedic method

The thoracolumbar rotation method, lumbar spine rotation method, and hyperextension thorax method are used when the patients are in the sitting position to correct the vertebral body rotation and thereby improve the Lateral curvature. (For specific operation methods and indications, contraindications, and precautions of the positive spine method, see Appendix B)

6.2.2.2 Traction and curvature adjusting

According to the type of scoliosis, the patients are treated with four – dimensional curvature adjusting therapy by chiropractic adjustment curvature traction bed based on the syndrome differentiation, in order to adjust the rotation and scoliosis of vertebral body and restore the physiological curvature of spine. (For specific operation methods, indications, contraindications, and precautions of traction and curvature adjusting method, see Appendix C) .

The above – mentioned therapy is performed once a day, 10 times a course, with a rest day, and then a second course, usually 4 – 6 courses are taken.

6.2.3 Drug therapy

6.2.3.1 Syndrome differentiation

6.2.3.1.1 Deficiency of kidney yang syndrome

Treatment: Tonifying kidney and invigorating yang.

Main formula: Modified yougui pill (*Jingyue Quanshu*) .

6.2.3.1.2 Kidney – spleen yang deficiency syndrome

Treatment: Warming the spleen and kidney.

Main formula: Modified shenqi pill (*Shanghan Lun*) plus fuzi lizhong pills(*Shanghan Lun*) .

6.2.3.1.3 Deficiency of kidney and blood stasis syndrome

Treatment: Tonifying kidney, invigorating the circulation of blood to remove the blood stasis.

Main formula: Modified gexia zhuyu tang(*Yilin Gaicuo*)

6.2.3.2 External medication

The traditional Chinese medicine plaster is applied to the chest and lumber concave side, to promote blood circulation and remove blood stasis, improve circulation and restore muscle strength. Commonly used "Qianshan Huoxue ointment"(SFDA approval number Z20025596) . See the plaster instructions for specific use.

6.2.3.3 Other medications

Improving bone metabolism and endocrine drugs can be used.

6.2.4 Exercise therapy

Use the sixth, thirteenth, fourteenth and fifteenth postures of the "Eighteen postures of strengthening the spine and body " for functional exercises to strengthen the functions of the back muscles and psoas major muscles to enhance their vitality and toughness, and maintain the balance of the spine inside and outside(Figure 1)

6.3 Efficacy evaluation

The efficacy evaluation has four classifications.

——Excellent: improvement of scoliosis is more than 30% .

——Good: improvement of scoliosis is between 10% and 29% .

——Poor: improvement of scoliosis is less than 10% .

——Invalid: no improvement in scoliosis.

6.4 Precautions

6.4.1　Bow in front and arrow in back posture. Pay attention to the convex lower limb in front and concave lower limb in back.

6.4.2　The muscle atrophy side is the main part in medicine ironing, acupuncture and massage.

6.4.3　The temperature is suitable for the patients when the patients are taking the ironing medicine thera-

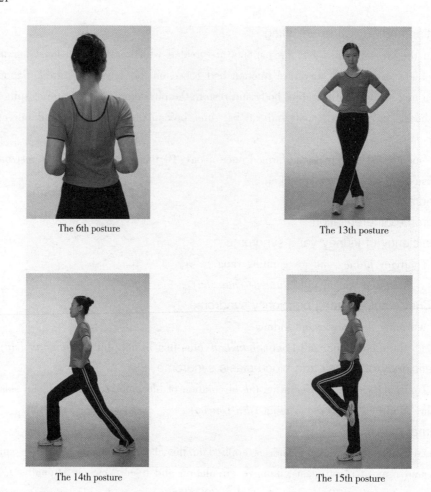

The 6th posture

The 13th posture

The 14th posture

The 15th posture

Figure1　The 6th posture, 13th posture, 14th posture, 15th posture of "Eighteen postures
of strengthening the spine and body"

py, so as to avoid scalding. Try to choose the drugs that are less irritating to the skin. If local skin has red spots and allergic reactions after ironing, it is necessary to stop using this method.

6.5　Contraindications

Spine – straightening method is given priority to rotation method, and violence is avoided by all means.

Appendix A

(Informative appendix)

Examination and diagnostic classification of adolescent idiopathic scoliosis

A. 1　Examination of adolescent idiopathic scoliosis

A. 1. 1　X – ray inspection

In the upright position of the spine, it can be seen that some spinous processes deviate from the midline, the spine protrudes to one side or both sides, some intervertebral spaces are unequal between left and right, the vertebral body is inclined, and both sides of the vertebral body are not equal in height. Cobb method can be used to measure the specific scoliosis angle. Abnormal physiological curvature of neck, chest and waist can be seen in lateral position.

Cobb method measurement: On the X – ray orthophoto, the convex upper and lower end vertebrae are determined firstly, and the upper and lower end plates of the main bend have the largest inclination to concave side, the upper end of the main bend is the upper end vertebra, and the lower end of the main bend is the lower end vertebra. Draw a flat line on the upper edge of the upper end vertebral body and the lower edge of the lower end vertebral body respectively, and make a vertical line on the two horizontal lines. The intersection angle of these two vertical lines is Cobb angle, and its specific degree can be measured by protractor. If the upper and lower edges of the final vertebra are unclear, the connection between the upper and lower edges of the pedicle can be taken, and then the intersection angle of the vertical lines is Cobb angle.

A. 1. 2　CT three – dimensional reconstruction of spine

Abnormal bone development can be clearly found.

A. 1. 2　Auxiliary inspection

Including height measurement, weight measurement, distance between fingertips in both arms outside the booth and other related items. The examinee bares the whole waist and back, stand naturally, the distance between his feet are as wide as the distance of his two shoulders, his eyes look at the front horizontally, his arms drop naturally, with palms inward. The examiner stands directly behind the patient and observes whether the shoulders of the examinee are symmetrical, whether the iliac crests on both sides are equal in height, and whether the spinous process connection deviates from the central axis. If more than one of the five items are abnormal, it can be diagnosed as torso asymmetry.

A. 2　Diagnostic classification

According to the anatomical position of the apex of the main curve of scoliosis, combined with clinical experience, adolescent idiopathic scoliosis can be divided into the following three types.

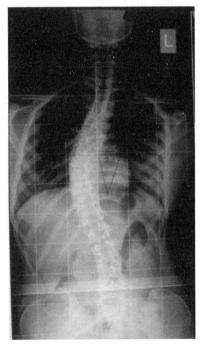

Figure A. 1　Thoracic vertebra single arc

A.2.1 Type Ⅰ

Thoracic vertebra single arc: The main arc is composed of thoracic vertebra, and the lumbar scoliosis is not obvious. The degree and prognosis of scoliosis are very different, and the radian can be developed to a very serious degree. Because of the rotation of vertebral body, the kyphosis of thoracic vertebra becomes flat, and the ribs rise backward, which leads to the decline of lung function, the corresponding symptoms such as chest tightness and shortness of breath occur. The degree of rib posterior bulge is not necessarily commensurate with the lateral convex angle(Figure A. 1).

Lumbar vertebra single arc: The main arc is composed of the lumbar spine. The thoracic scoliosis is not obvious, but it may cause the upper body to tilt sideways(Figure A. 2).

A.2.2 Type Ⅱ

Thoracic and lumbar vertebrae double arcs: The apex of thoracic vertebrae arc is at 7th thoracic segment and protrudes to the right, while the apex of lumbar vertebrae arc is at the first and second lumbar segments. Thoracic and lumbar scoliosis occur at the same time, with the same curvature. The convex shoulder rib bulges and the vertebral body rotates to the opposite side of the convex. There is no rotational deformity in the transitional vertebral body at the junction of thoracolumbar radian. Scoliosis tends to develop in adolescence (Figure A. 3).

A.2.3 Type Ⅲ

Cervicothoracic lumbar three arcs: Cervicothoracic segment, thoracic segment and lumbar segment appear scoliosis(Figure A. 4).

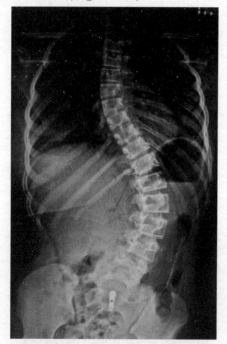

Figure A. 2　Lumbar vertebra single arc

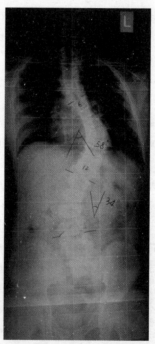

Figure A. 3　Thoracic and lumbar vertebrae double arcs

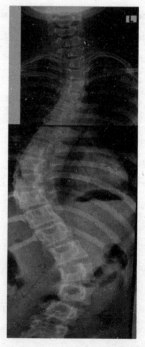

Figure A. 4　Cervicothoracic lumbar three arcs

Appendix B

(Informative appendix)

Common chiropractic manipulation and traction and curvature adjustment

B. 1　Chest lifting to hyperextension manipulation

B. 1. 1　Indications

Cervical disorders complicated with scoliosis of the thoracic vertebra, epiphyseal osteomalacia of the spine, arrhythmia of spinal origin, gastrointestinal dysfunction of spinal origin.

B. 1. 2　Contraindications

Severe osteoporosis.

B. 1. 3　Cautions

Don't over – exert knee pushing force.

B. 1. 4　Manipulation methods

[Method 1] Ask the patient to sit on the chiropractic chair, face the front, put the hands behind the neck with fingers of two hands crossing. The doctor stands behind the patient and pushes the upper thoracic vertebrae by one knee. Meanwhile, put the hands on the rib sides by passing over patient's shoulders and lift and pull the body back and up by holding the ribs of the patients.

[Method 2] Ask the patient to sit on the chiropractic chair, face the front, put the hands behind the neck with fingers of two hands crossing. The doctor stands behind the patient and oppositely holds patient's arms through armpits to lift and pull the body up. The doctor push the patient's chest by his own chest and lift and pull patient's body back and up by two hands.

[Method 3] Ask the patient to sit on the chiropractic chair, face the front, cross the arms in front of the chest and hold the shoulders by the hands. The doctor sits behind the patient and tries to broaden the scapulae by pulling patient's elbow joint of the opposite side through the armpit. At the same time, lift and pull the patient's body back and up.

B. 2　Thoracic and lumbar rotating manipulation

B. 2. 1　Indications

Disorder of thoracic and lumbar small joints, lumbar spondylolisthesis, prolapse of lumbar intervertebral disc, lumbar canal stenosis, scoliosis, irregular menstruation of spinal origin, osteoarthritis of lower limbs of spinal origin, gastrointestinal disorder of spinal origin, ankylosing spondylitis and spinal deformity.

B. 2. 2　Contraindications

After surgery on the thoracic and lumbar vertebra, severe osteoporosis of the lumbar vertebra, tumors of the thoracic and lumbar vertebra, tuberculosis of the thoracic and lumbar vertebra, myelitis of the thoracic and lumbar vertebra, being cautious for acute stage of prolapse of lumbar intervertebral disc, being cautious for patients with lumbar stiffness.

B. 2. 3　Cautions

Assistant is needed to fasten the hip. Do not blindly pursue the rotation sound by rotating repeatedly.

B. 2. 4　Manipulation methods

Ask the patient to sit on the chiropractic chair, face the front, put the hands behind the occipital region with fingers of two hands crossing, and bend forward slightly with the 12th thoracic vertebra and 1st lumbar vertebra as the supporting point. Take left deviation in spinous process for example, the assistant fastens the patient's right hip, while the practitioner stands at the left rear side, puts the left hand at the back of neck and chest (below DU14) by passing the front of left arm, and fastens the left of thoracolumbar joint of the patient by the right hand. The practitioner then rotates the patient's thoracolumbar region by the left hand. After the patient relaxes, exert opposite force of both hands quickly and simultaneously. In other words, rotate to the left by the left hand and push to the right by the right hand. Local bone sound can be heard. Manipulation on the right side is opposite to the left one.

B.3   Lumbar rotating manipulation

B.3.1   Indications

Dislocation of posterior lumbar joint, disorder of posterior lumbosacral joint, prolapse of lumbar intervertebral disc, lumbar canal stenosis, lumbar scoliosis.

B.3.2   Contraindications

B.3.2.1   Same to contraindications of the thoracic and lumbar rotating manipulation.

B.3.2.2   Patients with slipped vertebral disc compressing dural sac for more than a half are forbidden to use this method.

B.3.2.3   Patients with collapsed vertebral arch and spondylolisthesis should be cautious to use this method.

B.3.3   Cautions

Same to the cautions of the thoracic and lumbar rotating manipulation.

B.3.4 Manipulation methods

Ask the patient to sit on the chiropractic chair, face the front, put the hands behind the occipital region with fingers of two hands crossing, and bend forward with the affected spinous process as the supporting point. Take the left deviated spinous process for example, the assistant fastens the right hip, while the practitioner stands at the left rear side of the patient, puts the left hand on the right shoulder of the patient by crossing under the patient's left armpit, and fastens the left of the deviated spinous process by the right palm. The practitioner then shakes patient's waist and when the patient relaxes, exert opposite force of both hands quickly and simultaneously. In other words, rotate to the left by the left hand and push to the right by the right hand. Local bone sound can be heard. Manipulation on the right side is opposite to the left one.

B.4 Four – dimensional spinal curvature adjusting

B. 4.1 indications

B. 4.1.1   Flexion thoracolumbar fracture dislocation.

B. 4.1.2   Lumbar disc herniation with straightened curvature and reversed arch.

B. 4.1.3   Lumbar spinal stenosis with straightened curvature and reversed arch.

B. 4.1.4   Lumbar posterior joint malocclusion with straightened lumbar curvature and reversed arch.

B. 4.1.5   Scoliosis.

B. 4.1.6   lumbar spondylolisthesis with straightened, reversed arch or upper arch and lower arch lumbar curvature.

B. 4.2   Contraindication

B. 4.2.1   The diagnosis is not clear, and there is no X – ray diagnosis of bone and joint mechanical changes.

B. 4.2.2   In acute stage of lumbar disc herniation, the pain aggravated after traction.

B. 4.2.3   Patients with severe hypertension, heart disease, asthma and hyperthyroidism.

B. 4.2.4   Pregnant women and patients with severe osteoporosis.

B. 4.2.5   Patients after lumbar surgery.

B. 4.2.6   Patients with spinal tuberculosis, spinal osteomyelitis, spinal bone tumor, severe lower extremity osteoarthritis and severe varicose veins.

B. 4.3   Operation method

The patient lies on a chiropractic and curvature adjustment traction bed, and the upper body is placed over the armpit with a loop, and the lower limbs band are pulled at the upper and lower ends of the knee joints. The lower part of the body is lifted through a belt to a position that the chest and waist and the lower body are at an angle of $25° - 45°$ (Figure B. 1). Adjust the traction device to rise the lower limbs slowly. The lower body are suspended, and then the pallet is placed 30cm away from the lower limbs, it is advisable that the lower abdomen should leave the tray below. The angle of the lower limb and the traction bed is adjusted according to the lumbar curvature of the patient. Under normal circumstances, the fulcrum of the force acts on the joint of the thoracolumbar joint. Traction time is $20 - 30$ minutes, which is based on patient's tolerance. After the traction is removed, patients will rest in bed for $10 - 20$ minutes before going to the ground.

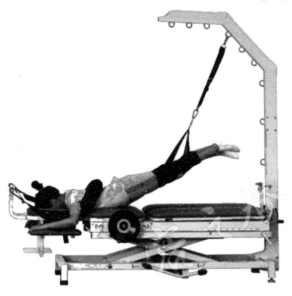

Figure B. 1   Four-dimensional spinal curvature adjusting

B. 4.4   Cautions

B. 4.4.1 The belt binding the lower limb can't be tied to the patella. The tightness should be suitable, avoiding too tight for blood circulation.

B. 4.4.2   Hanging traction of the lower limbs needs to be heightened little by little and patient's condition must be observed in the whole course.

B. 4.4.3   The traction duration should be tolerated by the patient and the traction time should be gradually increased.

B. 4.4.4   Pay close attention to the pulsation of the feet dorsal artery of the patient during the traction.

B. 4.4.5   Even and moderate removal of the traction is required and put down the supporting board slowly after disclosing the traction belt of the lower limbs.

图书在版编目（CIP）数据

国际中医临床实践指南青少年特发性脊柱侧凸症/世界中医药学会联合会 . —北京:中国中医药出版社,
2021. 11

ISBN 978 – 7 – 5132 – 7082 – 3

Ⅰ. ①青…　Ⅱ. ①世…　Ⅲ. ①青少年 – 脊柱畸形 – 中医治疗法 – 指南　Ⅳ. ①R274. 923 – 62

中国版本图书馆 CIP 数据核字（2021）第 146739 号

世界中医药学会联合会
国际中医临床实践指南青少年特发性脊柱侧凸症

*

中 国 中 医 药 出 版 社 出 版

北京经济技术开发区科创十三街 31 号院二区 8 号楼
邮政编码 100176
网址 www. cptcm. com
传真 010 64405721
廊坊市晶艺印务有限公司印刷
各地新华书店经销

*

开本 880 × 1230　1/16　印张 1.75　字数 47 千字
2021 年 11 月第 1 版　2021 年 11 月第 1 次印刷

*

书号 ISBN 978 – 7 – 5132 – 7082 – 3　定价 50.00 元

*

服务热线　010 – 64405510
购书热线　010 – 89535836
维权打假　010 – 64405753
微信服务号　zgzyycbs
微商城网址　https://kdt. im/LIdUGr
官方微博　http://e. weibo. com/cptcm
天猫旗舰店网址　https://zgzyycbs. tmall. com

世界中医药学会联合会

国际中医临床实践指南青少年特发性脊柱侧凸症

SCM 0059—2021

*

中国中医药出版社出版

北京经济技术开发区科创十三街31号院二区8号楼

邮政编码 100176

网址 www.cptcm.com

传真 010-64405721

廊坊市晶艺印务有限公司印刷

各地新华书店经销

*

开本 880×1230 1/16 印张1.75 字数 47千字

2021年11月第1版 2021年11月第1次印刷

*

书号 ISBN 978-7-5132-7082-3 定价50.00元

*

网址 www.cptcm.com

服务热线 010-64405510

购书热线 010-89535836

维权打假 010-64405753

微信服务号 zgzyycbs

微商城网址 https://kdt.im/LIdUGr

官方微博 http://e.weibo.com/cptcm

天猫旗舰店网址 https://zgzyycbs.tmall.com

如有印装质量问题请与本社出版部联系（010-64405510）

ISBN 978-7-5132-7082-3

9 787513 270823 >